Msc Krzysztof Klimek

How to start living without pain, in easy steps.

Photographs: BlueSky Pixels, Joanna Klimek

Editing: Krzysztof Klimek, Joanna Klimek, Mariola Piotrowska

Copyright © 2021 Klimek Academy Ltd.

Contents

Preface 7
Part I 11
  Restoration of movement ranges in the hips 11
  Physical exercises 11
    1. Child pose 12
    2. Seated forward bend 13
    3. "Open" seat 14
    4. Seated scissors 15
    5. Knee – chest 17
    6. Knee – chest (opposite side) 18
    7. "Frog" 19
    8. Cross-legged pose 20
    9. Half lotus 21
    10. Easy twist 22
    11. "Mountain" pose 22
    12. "Japanese" bow 24
    13. "Dog" 25
    14. Back kick 26
  Chair sitting positions 27

Part II 29
Restoration of movement ranges in the lumbar 29
spine 29
Base positions 30
1. "90/90" 31
2. "Three arches" pose 32
3. Prone position 33
4. "Child" pose 34
5. Recovery position 35
Physical exercises 36
1. "Sphinx" 36
2. "Cobra" 38
3. "Cobra with a twist" 39
4. "Prone lying scissors" 40
5. "The bow" 41
6. "Cat cow pose" 42
7. "Cat cow pose on forearms" 43
8. "Puppy" 44
9. "Knee – chest" 45
10. "Knees – chest" 46
11. "Diagonal knee" 47
12. "Twist" 48

13. "Russian man" 49
Myofascial trigger points of the lumbar region.......................**50**
Part III **51**
Restoring balance in the thoracic spine **51**
Base positions **53**
    1. "Arrow" 53
    2. "Crucified" 54
    3. "The half moon" 55
Physical exercises **56**
    1. "Dead man" 56
    2. "Dry swimming" 57
    3. "Cat cow on elevation" 58
    4. "Shoulder fall" 61
    5. "Side bend on the chair" 62
    6. "Chair twist" 63
    7. "Straighten up on the chair" 64
    8. "Wings" 65
Part IV **66**
Restoring balance in the cervical spine **66**
Base positions **68**
    1. "Balanced position" 68
    2. "Side position" 69

Physical exercises 70
    1. "Tik Tok" 70
    2. "No" 71
    3. "The sulk" 72
    4. "Chin – sternum" 73
    5. "Deeper Tik Tok" 74
    6. "Deeper bend forward" 75
The end 76

Healing the body through movement

Postural positions, exercises, relaxation

Preface

A balanced body is a healthy body

In this book I will present the possibilities and methods of balancing a human body. Balance can be obtained by introducing healthy movement, breathing and eating habits.

This programme is based on the many years of my clinical practice. During my work, I have understood that the only way to completely heal the dysfunctions of locomotive organs, and the pain that is a result of such dysfunctions, is through a holistic psychophysical approach. It is important to consider an evolutionary change of movement habits, eating habits and mental habits, as well as the learning process and cultivation of mental and physical relaxation. Relearning the correct and effective breathing patterns is the only effective and long-lasting form of real selfhealing. The role of the therapist in this system is not treating the patient in the common sense of the word. The therapist has to indicate the right path and support the process of self-healing in the patient. Such an approach leads to the growth of self-awareness in the patient which allows them not to be dependent on any treatment. A healthy lifestyle becomes the natural way of living for the patient. This allows them to make conscious decisions that keep their body healthy.

If other treatment techniques, e.g. chiropractic, are conducted correctly, they are effective "painkillers" that reduce or remove the physical pain for a limited amount of time. However, they do not remove the real causes of the pain. Such methods also turn out not to be very effective from a long-term perspective.

I used such treatment techniques for a few years and my practice was thriving. However, after three or four years some of the patients were coming back with the same problems or even in a worse condition than before. Some of them told me, "Your techniques helped me for some time but eventually the pain keeps coming back." That led to a therapeutic crisis in my career. I started looking for different solutions and methods that would complete my practice. I became a student of the best-known therapists, lecturers and therapeutic methods around the world. At the same time, I was deepening my philosophy with a study of Chinese medicine and Ayurveda.
I travelled to Central and Latin America to learn and work with people of native cultures where I became familiar with natural healing methods. All of those experiences showed me one common point. Everything we do should lead to BALANCE.

Lack of balance reveals itself in the physical and psychological spheres. Those spheres are inseparable.

Everything is mental and the mental expression manifests itself in the physical form. The physical body is the manifestation of personality integration. Breathing patterns and muscle structure are the psycho-spiritual manifestation. These reflect on the way and quality of our social existence. They express the balance or lack of it.

Balance disorder is the result of the negative personality stimulation (lack of movement in peripheral range of movement, static muscle overload, e.g. staying in a sitting or standing position for a long time, or repeating the same movement for a long time) and lack of psycho-spiritual hygiene (chronic stress, media overuse, lack of relationship with times of the day and seasons, lack of connection with the emotions, judging) and lack of nutritional hygiene. For example, relaxation while watching television does not provide enough movement or oxygen to our body. It often negatively stimulates our emotional system as well.

The results of lack of balance show in different parts of the body:

- head, face, temporomandibular joints
- neck, superior thoracic aperture
- shoulders, arms, hands
- thoracic spine, ribs, sternum, diaphragm
- lumbar spine, stomach
- pelvis, hips, thighs, knees, feet

The most common conditions are lower back pain, neck pain, hip pain, shoulder pain, sciatica, brachialgia, headache, knee pain, "jaw clicking", pain between shoulder

blades, pain under shoulder blades, dizziness, balance disorder, stomach ache, painful menstruations.
We cannot find an unambiguous cause of organic disease (e.g. bone fracture, cancerous lump, etc.) in the objective research.

Restoring BALANCE happens through recognising the current body posture and functional limitations.

At the beginning we find the area that is mostly affected by chronic stress and the patterns of reacting to stress. Then, we learn how to quickly recognise the lack of balance symptoms. Prognostic pains are usually the type of pain that appeared before but there was a belief it would go away, or, for example, we feel shoulder pain for some time but it stopped and we do not start a therapy to find out where the pain comes from.

It is important to learn how to quickly recognise the lack of balance symptoms, e.g., prognostic pains (usually the type of pain that appeared before but there was a belief it would go away, or we felt pain that went away after a while so we did not start a therapy to find out its cause)

Next, we adjust the individual process of myofascial stimulation, connected to re-creation of breathing patterns (e.g. diaphragmatic), relaxation learning, restoration of deep sensation, introduction of healthy eating habits and formation of movement patterns.

Part I

Restoration of movement ranges in the hips

Sedentary lifestyle (e.g. incorrect chair position, lack of feet grounding, lack of stomach breathing pattern) or premature potty training for babies and infants below two years of age result in a physical balance disorder that leads to degenerative hip disease.

Lack of balance in the psychophysical sphere is the result of introverted nature, stubbornness, toughness towards oneself, fierceness, and lack of care for one's own needs by common fulfilment of the needs of others.

Physical exercises

Gradual restoration of balance happens through the recovery of the physiological range of movement in the joints, normalisation of muscular tensions, strengthening of stabiliser muscles and the formation of positive movement habits. An appropriate level of body hydration is also an important aspect. We never cross the pain boundary while developing movement ranges.

It is recommended that you drink two glasses of water before the exercises.

1. Child pose

Exercise description: Kneeling position (you can use a blanket or a soft cushion under the knees, if needed), chest bent down, forehead touching the floor (or cushion), arms lying along the torso, the back of the hands touching the floor, palms directed towards the feet.

During the exercise, you need to concentrate on calm, diaphragmatic breathing. Exercise duration should be 3 to 5 minutes.

Goal: Hip muscles and lower spine stretch, reduction of nervous system tension and mental relaxation.

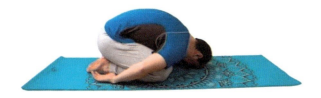

2. Seated forward bend

Exercise description: Sit on the ground with your legs slightly apart, and place a yoga roller or a rolled blanket underneath your knees for support. Next, bend forward with your knees facing outward, your belly positioned between the knees and your palms placed on the lower leg (you can also grab your ankles, if possible). Inhale with a conscious belly movement outward and then exhale with a belly movement inward. On the exhale, bend your body forward slightly deeper, on the inhale, relax the stretch.

Exercise duration should be 1 to 3 minutes.

Goal: Forward bend range deepening, hip joint relaxation and activation of diaphragmatic breathing pattern.

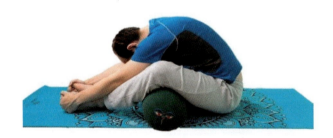

3. "Open" seat

Exercise description: Sit against the wall. If it is painful or not possible, sit on a folded blanket or cushion so that your pelvis is lifted. Soles of feet touching together, knees facing outward, put your heels as close to the pelvis as possible, keep your back straight, against the wall.

Movement: On the exhale, open your hips, and the knees drop to the floor. Pull your heels toward the pelvis. On the exhale, relax your body.

Repeat the exercise for 5 to 10 breaths.

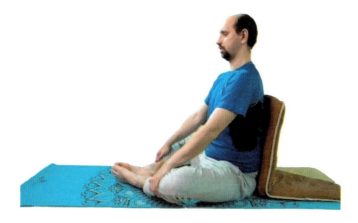

4. Seated scissors

Exercise description: Sit against the wall, keep your pelvis next to the wall (if it is painful or not possible, sit on a folded blanket or cushion so that your pelvis is lifted), legs together and straight out in front of you. Keep your knees straight and "active" feet (toes pointing upward).

Movement: Make a slow straddle stretch to the maximum of your ability and move your legs back together. Repeat 10 times.

Movement range development: Legs wide open, deep inhale with a belly movement outward and exhale with a belly movement inward. On the exhale deepen the straddle, on the inhale, relax.

Repeat the exercise for 5 to 10 breaths.

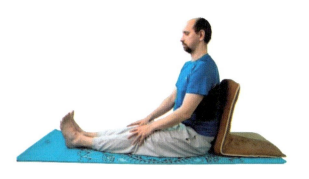

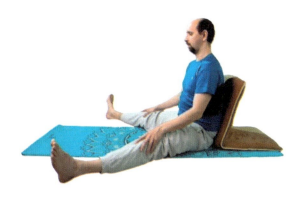

5. Knee – chest

Exercise description: Lie down on your back, bend one of the legs and use your hands to pull it towards your chest. Keep the second leg straight, both feet "active" (toes pointing upward).

Movement: Pull the knee toward chest on the same side of the body. On the exhale, deepen the movement by pulling the knee toward the chest and extend the straightened leg. On the inhale, extend the spine and drop the pelvis to the floor.

Repeat the exercise for 5 to 10 breaths on each side of the body.

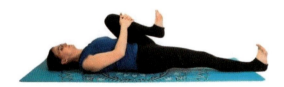

6. Knee – chest (opposite side)

Exercise description: Lie down on your back, bend one of your legs and use your hands to pull it towards your chest. Keep the second leg straight, both feet "active" (toes pointing upward).

Movement: Pull the knee to the chest toward the opposite side of the body. On the exhale, deepen the movement of pulling, on the inhale, extend the spine and straightened leg.

Repeat the exercise for 5 to 10 breaths on each side of the body.

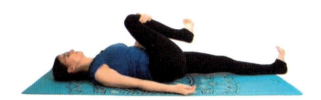

7. "Frog"

Exercise description: Lie down on your back, pull both knees toward the chest and grab your feet with your hands. Keep the spine and pelvis "attached to the floor".

Movement: On the exhale, open the hips and straighten up your knees. On the inhale, relax your legs.
Repeat the exercise for 5 to 10 breaths.

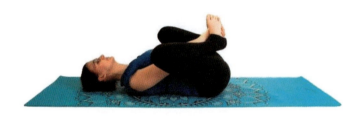

8. Cross-legged pose

Exercise description: Sit on the sitting bones with your legs crossed, straight spine, and hands on your knees. If you have substantial movement limitations, you can use knee support. Halfway through the exercise, cross your legs the other way.

Movement: On the exhale, your hands press the knees toward the floor. On the inhale, relax the legs and stretch the spine upward.

Repeat the exercise for 5 to 10 breaths.

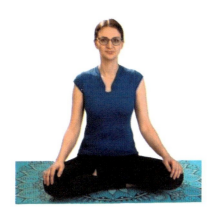

9. Half lotus

Exercise description: Bend your left leg and put it on the floor with your heel pulled towards the opposite side buttock. Put your right leg on top of the left, keeping the right foot on the left knee. Keep the spine straight, hands resting on the knees. Swap the legs' position halfway through the exercise.

Movement: On the exhale, press your hands on the knees, straightening the spine. On the inhale, relax the pose.

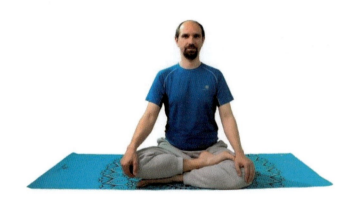

10. Easy twist

Exercise description: Straighten your left leg and rest it on the floor. Place the foot of your right leg next to the knee of the left leg (outer side) and twist your body towards the right. Shift your left arm across and rest the elbow behind the right knee. Place the other hand on the floor behind your back for support.

Movement: On the exhale, deepen the rotation, and on the inhale pull the spine upward.

Repeat the exercise for 5 to 10 breaths.

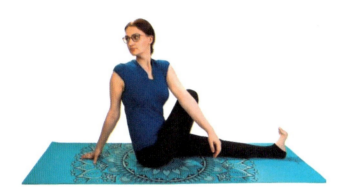

11. "Mountain" pose

Exercise description: Sit back on the heels. Keep your knees together, spine straight and hands resting on your thighs. If you feel pain in your feet, you can put a blanket or cushion underneath. However, if you feel knee pain, you can either put a cushion underneath your buttocks or sit on a yoga roller.

Movement: On the exhale, pull the spine upward, and on the inhale relax the pose.

Repeat the exercise for 5 to 10 breaths.

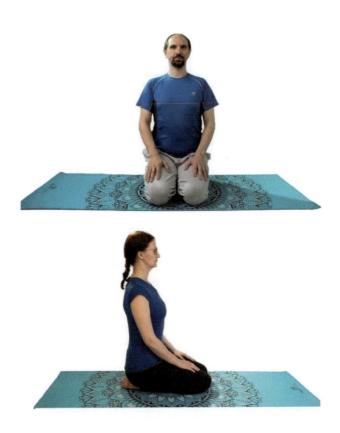

12. "Japanese" bow

Exercise description: Sit back onto the heels, keep your big toes together and your knees apart. Bend the torso forward and pull your arms above the head with the palms facing downward.

Movement: On the exhale stretch the back, extending your arms at the same time. Keep your buttocks on top of the heels. On the inhale, make an outward belly movement and relax the pose.

Repeat the exercise for 5 to 10 breaths.

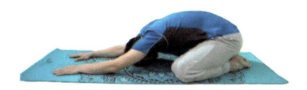

13. "Dog"

Exercise description: All fours pose, head facing the floor.
Movement: On the exhale, raise one of the legs to the side. On the inhale, come back to the all fours pose and then change the leg.

Repeat the exercise 5 to 10 times for each leg.

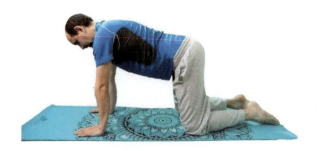

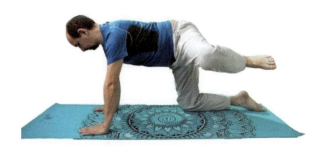

14. Back kick

Exercise description: Standing position, hands on the hips.
Movement: On the inhale make a circle with your leg towards the back. On the exhale, the leg comes back to the starting position.

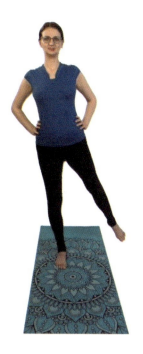

Chair sitting positions

Incorrect sitting positions. We often place our legs under the chair or we cross them. In that position, our back is bent. This position makes breathing difficult and causes hamstring muscles contracts.

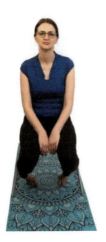
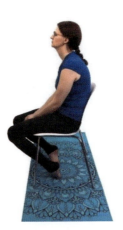

Correct sitting position. Sole of the feet positioned on the floor. Knees bent at around 90 degrees, the bend angle of the hips also around 90 degrees. Keep your back straight and the head straight on top of the spine.

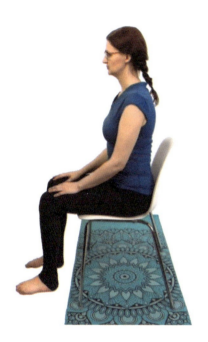

Part II

Restoration of movement ranges in the lumbar spine

Balance disorder in the lumbar part of the spine is the result of physical overload in this area, such as:
incorrect standing position or sedentary lifestyle and lack of appropriate physical activity during the day. On the other hand, there is also the emotional aspect, which has an impact on the balance disorder in this part of the spine.

Common causes of this are: encouraging babies to walk too early, putting pressure and having expectations toward a teenager (e.g. we expect teenagers to be strong and physically active). Such attitudes lead to stability disorders in the economical, family or professional spheres.
Disorders in the sexual sphere are also another significant cause of lack of balance in the lumbar spine. Some of these are excessive masturbation, watching pornography and having sexual contacts without the internal agreement with ourselves.

We need to remember that the spine is one connected column and whatever happens in one part of it has its result in another. However, for the didactic purposes of this book, I decided to divide the exercises according to spine parts.

Physical exercises allow the restoration of the physiological movement range in the spine joints, muscle flexibility and strength of the stabiliser muscles. In order to regain balance, it is very important to restore the natural breathing pattern. It decreases the pressure in the abdominal cavity significantly and normalises the movement of intestines and other internal organs at the same time.

Weight control and appropriate body hydration are the basic factors that support balance restoration. Diet should mainly be based on reducing the substances which intensify inflammation in the body. These are: "spicy" dishes, "heavy" food in a mainly meat-based diet, sweets, and drinks that accelerate dehydration, e.g. coffee, energy drinks or alcohol.

Base positions

The below positions are especially recommended in the sharp pain phase.

1. "90/90"

Description: Lie down and bend the hips at 90 degrees. Place a chair or cushions under the lower legs so that your knees are bent at 90 degrees. Place your hands along the body, palms directed toward the hips, palms facing upward. Breathe activating the "abdominal track", which means you push the belly outward on the inhale and pull it in on the exhale.

Stay in this position for 30 minutes to 2 hours (depending on the pain level).

Return from this position slowly, turning on the side, and removing your legs one by one.

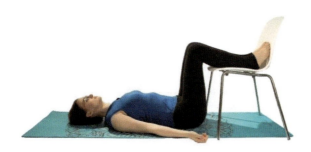

2. "Three arches" pose

Description: Lying on the back, put a small roller (around 10 cm) under the knees. Next, put a small roller (5 to 10 cm depending on the physiological body structure) under the lumbar region and then create the third arch by placing a roller (around 10 cm) under the neck. The rollers should be made of soft material: you could use, for example, rolled-up towels or blankets.

Activate the "abdominal track" (see "90/90" exercise).

Stay in this position for 30 minutes to 2 hours and return from this position slowly through the side.

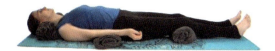

3. Prone position

Description: Place a roller (around 20 cm) on the level of the ankles, put a cushion under the belly and pelvis and place your hands under your forehead so that you can keep your head straight and breathe freely.

Activate the "abdominal track" (see "90/90" exercise).

Stay in this position for 30 minutes to 1 hour.

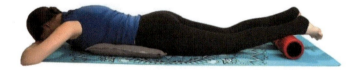

4. "Child" pose

Description: Kneeling position, torso bent forward as much as possible, forehead rests on the floor. If you cannot touch the floor with your forehead, please put a cushion under your head. Place your hands along the body, palms directed towards the hips, palms facing upward.

Stay in this position for 5 to 30 minutes.

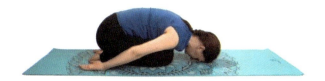

5. Recovery position

Description: Lie down on the side with the bottom leg slightly bent and the upper leg bent in the hip and knee at 90 degrees. Place a roller under the upper leg so that the pelvis is positioned at 90 degrees. The upper part of the torso remains straight with your head on the cushion so that you can keep your spine straight (head is the extension of the spine).

This position is recommended for sleeping.

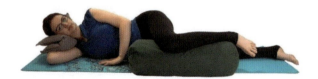

Physical exercises

All the exercises should be performed slowly and within your painless movement range. If you start feeling pain at any point, you need to change the movement direction.

1. "Sphinx"

Exercise description: Lie prone with your forearms rested on the floor at the level of the chest, elbows close to the body. On the exhale, raise the chest up, head looking at the ceiling and the neck making an arch. Keep the position 5 to 10 seconds. On the inhale, come back to the lying prone position.

Repeat the exercise 10 to 20 times.

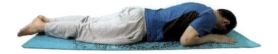

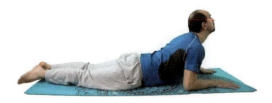

2. "Cobra"

Exercise description: Prone position, hands positioned at the level of the shoulders. On the exhale, raise your body upwards making your elbows as straight as possible. Head directed toward the ceiling, neck makes an arch.
Stay in this position for 5 to 10 seconds. On the inhale, come back to the prone position.

Repeat this exercise 10 to 20 times.

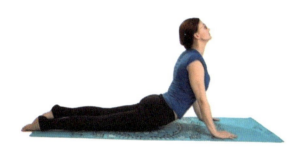

3. "Cobra with a twist"

Exercise description: Prone position with one arm leaning against the forearm and next to the torso, the other arm leaning on the palm at the level of the shoulder. On the exhale, straighten out the elbow of the hand leaning on the palm. Turn your head towards the arm leaning against the forearm. On the inhale, come back to the prone position.

Repeat this exercise, going as far as you can, 10 times on each side (stop movement at the pain boundary).

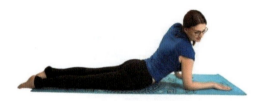

4. "Prone lying scissors"

Exercise description: Prone position. We pull our hands above the head keeping the arms straight. On the exhale, raise one of the legs up. Stay in this position for 5 to 10 seconds. On the inhale, come back to the prone position.

Repeat this exercise 10 times on each leg.

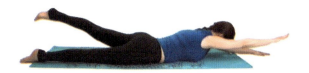

5. "The bow"

Exercise description: Kneeling position, big toes touching together and knees wide apart (the ground should be soft so that you do not feel any pain in your feet). If your body does not allow you to perform the full kneeling position, then you should put a cushion or a soft roller under your bottom. Bend your body forward and rest your hands on the floor in this position. On the exhale, deepen the body bend. On the inhale, relax the tension.

Maintain the movement for 1 to 3 minutes.

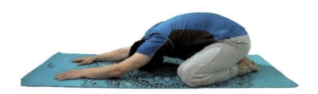

6. "Cat cow pose"

Exercise description: Front support position, in other words "all fours pose".
On the exhale, raise your back up (picture: position 1), pulling in the belly at the same time. Stay in this position for up to 5 seconds. Next, on the inhale, lower the back and relax the belly (picture: position 2).

Repeat this exercise 10 to 20 times.

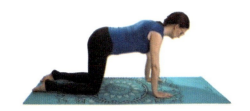

Starting position

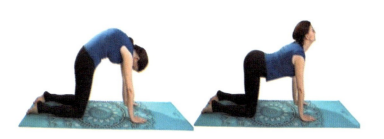

Position 1   Position 2

7. "Cat cow pose on forearms"

Exercise description: Front support position with arms bent at the elbows, forearms resting on the floor. On the exhale, raise the back up, pulling the belly in at the same time (picture: position 1). Stay in this position for up to 5 seconds. On the inhale, lower the back and relax the belly (picture: position 2).

Repeat this exercise 10 to 20 times.

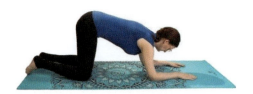

Starting position

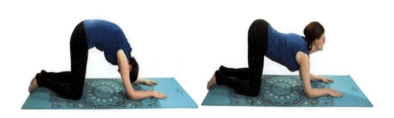

Position 1   Position 2

8. "Puppy"

Exercise description: Front support position. On the exhale, bend your body to the side, head looking at your bottom. Stay in this position for up to 5 seconds. On the inhale, come back to the starting position. Repeat the same movement on the other side of the body. Repeat this exercise 10 times on each side.

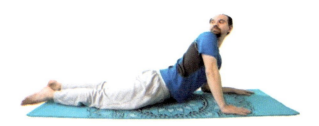

9. "Knee – chest"

Exercise description: Lie on your back. Keep one leg straight with an active foot (toes pointing upward). Bend the other leg at the knee and pull it toward your belly (active foot). Place both your hands on the bent leg. On the exhale, pull the knee toward your chest harder. On the inhale, relax the tension. Repeat this exercise 5 to 10 times on each leg.

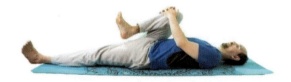

10. "Knees – chest"

Exercise description: Lie on your back. Bend both legs at the knees and pull them toward the chest. Grab each leg at the knees and pull them apart slightly. On the exhale, pull the knees toward the chest harder. On the inhale, relax the tension.

Repeat the exercise 5 to 10 times.

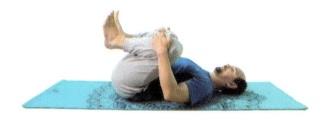

11. "Diagonal knee"

Exercise description: Lie on your back. Keep one of the legs straight with an active foot. Bend the other leg at the knee and pull it toward the opposite side of your chest. On the exhale, pull the knee harder. On the inhale, relax the tension.

Repeat this exercise 10 times on each leg.

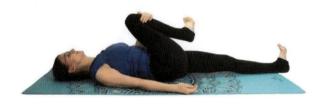

12. "Twist"

Exercise description: Lie on your back. Bend both legs at the knees with your feet together. Place your arms wide apart at the level of your chest. On the exhale, drop your knees to the side and stay in this position for about 5 seconds. On the inhale, come back to the starting position.

Repeat this exercise 10 times on each side.

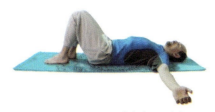

Initial position

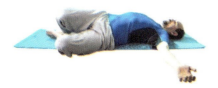

Position after movement

13. "Russian man"

Exercise description : Lie down on your back and bend both legs at the knees. Place one leg on top of the other and lean the lateral ankle against the knee of the other leg. Grab the thigh of the first leg with your hands.

On the exhale, pull the knee of the first leg toward the chest and position the hip of the other leg in the outward position. Stay in this position for up to 5 seconds. On the inhale, extend the spine, and "attach" the sacrum bone to the floor.

Repeat this exercise 5 to 10 times on each leg.

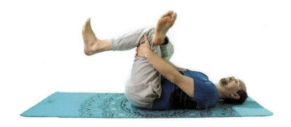

Myofascial trigger points of the lumbar region

The most effective myofascial trigger points (the points that reduce pain, and relax muscles and ligaments) for the lumbar region are located in the area of the posterior superior iliac spine (the points that stick out the most at the back of the pelvis next to the spine). We often feel the palpatory tissue changes in this area.

Compression technique consists of pressing the point that is the most painful. We make a circular movement around that point. The movement is on the boundary of "bearable" or "pleasant" pain.
We keep the pressure until the pain starts decreasing to the level that it can be barely felt.

This technique is recommended in the prone position. On the exhale, we increase the pressure slightly. On the inhale, we decrease the pressure level.

Part III

Restoring balance in the thoracic spine

The key to restoring balance in the thoracic spine is the correlation with the breathing mechanism and the relationship with "the neighbours", which are the ribs, lumbar spine and the cervical spine. Lack of balance in this area mainly shows the ineffective breathing pattern.
Its main role is to protect and support the two main body organs – lungs and heart. One of the most important muscles in our body, which is the diaphragm, is attached to the root of the thoracic spine.

The diaphragm takes a more or less active part in the breathing process and it also passively supports digestion. It divides the body into the lower and upper part. The biggest body channels such as the aorta, vena cava and alimentary canal run through the diaphragm.

The diaphragm is closely related to the emotional state. If there is tension or functional changes in the diaphragm, they lead the body into mechanisms typical for extreme emotional states, such as fear or anger.
Achieving full balance in the thoracic spine allows one to quickly get control over emotional state changes and automatic body reactions, such as "fight and fly" or "rest and digest". As a result of lack of balance in the thoracic spine, the body works within the above patterns even though there is no need for them and it disturbs its general

balance at the same time. It is mainly the ability to adopt and transport oxygen that is disturbed.

The main factors that have an impact on lack of balance in this region of the spine are: incorrect sitting position, obesity, general lack of movement or smoking. Psychologically, it reflects the lack of openness to new things, anxiety, emotional wounds, low self-esteem, and vocal expression disorders.

Physical exercises allow the restoration of an effective breathing pattern, and an effective oxygen exchange in the body. They improve the proprioception in the body. They also make the digestive process more efficient and build up awareness of the emotional states.

Base positions

1. "Arrow"

Exercise description: Prone position with the arms straight and extended above the head. On the exhale, stretch the body. On the inhale, relax the position. Engage your belly in the breathing process. When you take a breath, pull the belly in. On the exhale, pull the belly out. Stay in this position from 1 to 10 minutes while breathing slowly.

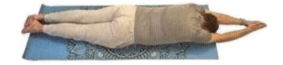

2. "Crucified"

Exercise description: Lie on your back with your hands extended to the sides. Put a large roller (10-20 cm) under the thoracic spine, and place a cushion under your head so that it does not tilt back too much. On the exhale, pull in the belly. On the inhale, push out the belly. Stay in this position from 1 to 10 minutes.

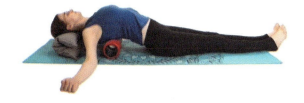

3. "The half moon"

Exercise description: Lie down on the side and place the arm you're lying on in a way that is comfortable for you. Extend the other arm above the head keeping the elbow straight. Keep your legs straight in the knees and hips. On the exhale, stretch the body. On the inhale, relax the tension.

Stay in this position from 1 to 10 minutes.

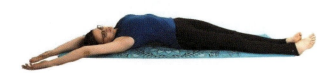

Physical exercises

1. "Dead man"

Exercise description: Lie down on your back. Keep your arms alongside your body with palms facing upwards. Inhale pushing your belly out and exhale pulling your belly in. This position is designed to relax and oxygenate your body.

Repeat it for 20 breaths.

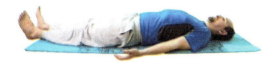

2. "Dry swimming"

Exercise description: Prone position with your hands extended above the head. On the inhale, pull your elbows toward the side of your torso and raise your head above the ground. Hold your breath and count to 5. On the exhale, lift your hands above the head, hold your breath and count to 5.

Repeat the cycle from 10 to 15 times.

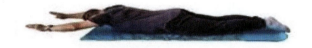

3. "Cat cow on elevation"

Exercise description: Front support position with your hands on the roller (around 20 cm diameter).

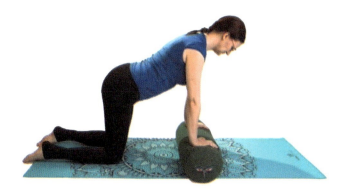

A) On the exhale, make a spine movement upwards. On the inhale, lower your spine down. Repeat the exercise 20 times in each direction.

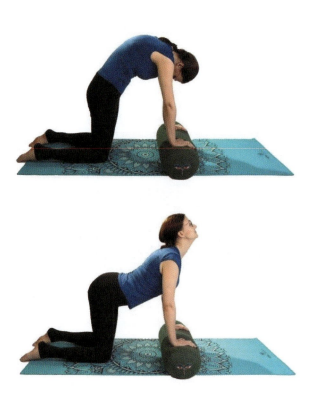

B) On the exhale, raise one arm up to the side. On the inhale, come back to the starting position. Repeat the exercise 10 times on each side.

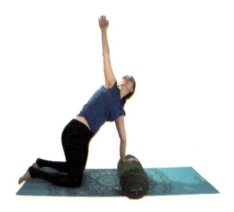

C) On the exhale, turn to one side. On the inhale, come back to the centre. Repeat the exercise 10 times on each side.

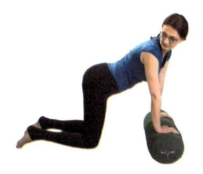

4. "Shoulder fall"

Exercise description: On all fours position. On the exhale, move your left arm along the floor towards the right so that your left shoulder rests on the floor. On the inhale, come back to the centre. Repeat the exercise 10 times on each side.

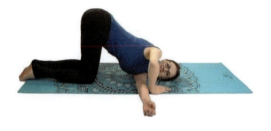

#

5. "Side bend on the chair"

Exercise description: Sit on the chair, keeping both feet stable on the floor and your back rested on the back of the chair. On the exhale, bend your body to the side, the arm on that side of the body sliding down. On the inhale, come back to the centre.

Repeat the exercise 10 times on each side.

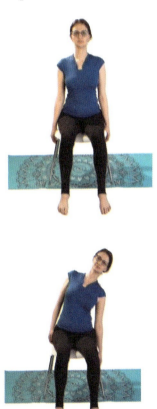

6. "Chair twist"

Exercise description: Sit on the chair and rest your back on the back of the chair. Keep your feet stable on the floor. On the exhale, turn your body to the left and grab the right side of the chair with your left hand, and the left side of the chair with your right hand. On the inhale, extend your spine. On the exhale, intensify the rotation.

Repeat the exercise 10 times on each side.

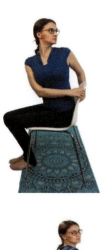

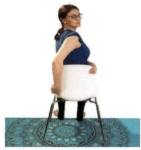

7. "Straighten up on the chair"

Exercise description: Sit on the chair, keeping your feet stable on the floor. On the inhale, tilt your back backward. On the exhale, relax the body.

Repeat the exercise from 10 to 15 times.

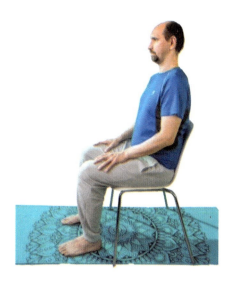

8. "Wings"

Exercise description: Stand up, keeping your arms straight and hands together, and place them in front of your chest. On the inhale, open your chest by shifting your arms to the sides. On the exhale, move the arms back and touch hands in front of the chest.

Repeat this movement dynamically from 10 to 20 times.

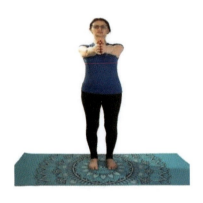

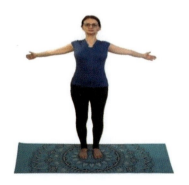

Part IV

Restoring balance in the cervical spine

Restoring the balance in the cervical spine is the basic condition for the right functioning of our brain. A balanced cervical spine allows the delivery of a sufficient amount of blood to the brain and ensures the transmission of the correct nerve impulses. Its functionality has a great impact on the provision of balance to your whole body. The cervical spine "carries" the head, for which it plays the role of a support.

The body tries to stay in balance by keeping the eyeline parallel to the horizon at all times. Psychologically, the neck "carries all the problems that the head is loaded with". It is also the main tool to navigate our awareness. There is a significant link between the neck's functionality and our ability to change the way we look at things and our visual range.

Overload in the cervical spine is typical for people who worry too much. They take on too much responsibility or look away from certain areas in their life – not wanting to see it. Lack of balance in this region is often related to deep depression and fear.

We distinguish a few basic neck and head positions. For example, we can come across terms such as "the noose", which is characterised by the head tilted to the side. It looks like the hanged man, or "tortoise" when the neck is short and the head hidden between the shoulders.

Physical exercises allow the restoration of the myofascial-skeletal balance. The head achieves a more stable support and natural movement ranges that are physiologically quite large in this region, in comparison to the rest of the spine. They allow the correct oxygenation and blood supply. Balance in this part also provides the correctness and clarity of mental processes.

Base positions

1. "Balanced position"

Exercise description: Lie down on your back. Rest your head on a small cushion or in case of significant disorders in the cervical spine, use an orthopaedic cushion Place your arms alongside the torso with your palms facing upward.

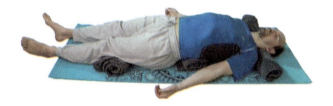

2. "Side position"

Exercise description: Lie down on the side and place your head so that it is an extension of the spine.

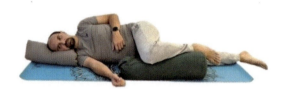

Physical exercises

Please perform each exercise slowly and within your (painless) body limits.

1. "Tik Tok"

Exercise description: Lie down on your back. On the exhale, bend your head to the shoulder. On the inhale, come back to the starting position. Repeat the exercise on the other side of the body.

Repeat the exercise 10 times on each side.

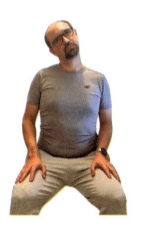 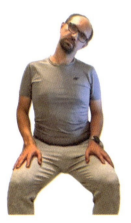

2. "No"

Exercise description: Lie down on your back. On the exhale, turn your head to one side. On the inhale, come back to the centre.

Repeat the exercise 10 times on each side.

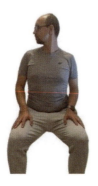 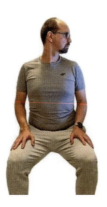

3. "The sulk"

Exercise description: Lie down on your back. On the exhale, turn your neck to one side, and direct your sight upward and to the back, simultaneously.

We repeat the exercise 10 times on each side.

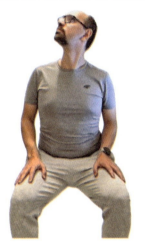
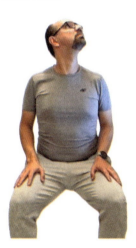

4. "Chin – sternum"

Exercise description: Lie down on your back. On the exhale, bring your chin closer to the sternum without lifting your head off the ground. On the inhale, relax the position.

Repeat the exercise from 10 to 20 times.

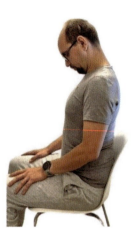

5. "Deeper Tik Tok"

Exercise description: Sit down on a chair with your back rested on the back of the chair and your feet fully flat on the floor. On the inhale, grab your head with one hand and bend your head to the side. On the exhale, relax the position. Take another breath in and intensify the bend (by pulling your head to the side with your hand).
Repeat the exercise for 5 breaths on each side.

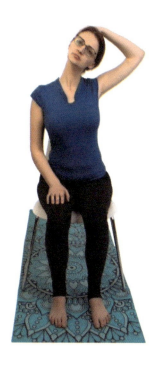

6. "Deeper bend forward"

Exercise description: Sit down on a chair with your back straight and your feet flat on the floor. Place both of your hands on the back of the head. On the exhale, bend your head forward deeper. On the inhale, relax the tension.

Repeat this exercise 10 times.

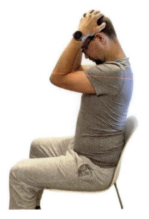

The end

In this book, we presented a few sets of exercises that are extremely effective in reducing pain and improving the mobility of your joints.

Paying attention to the way we breathe while we exercise is the unique part of these sets. It is one of the tips that is lacking most in other publications of this type. This makes them ineffective and discourages people from continuing with the programme.

We wish you effective exercising and getting rid of the pain!!!

Printed in Great Britain
by Amazon